T0193917

Metamorfit

Renewing Your Mind, Reshaping Your Body

DONALD STEVENS JR.

WESTBOW
PRESS®
A DIVISION OF THOMAS NELSON
& ZONDERVAN

Scripture taken from the King James Version of the Bible.

Scripture quotations marked NIV are taken from the Holy Bible, New
International Version. NIV. Copyright 1973, 1978, 1984 by International
Bible Society. Used by permission of Zondervan. All rights reserved.

Scripture quotations marked AMP are from The Amplified Bible, Old
Testament copyright 1965, 1987 by the Zondervan Corporation. The
Amplified Bible, New Testament copyright 1954, 1958, 1987 by The
Lockman Foundation. Used by permission. All rights reserved.

WestBow Press books may be ordered through booksellers or by contacting:

WestBow Press
A Division of Thomas Nelson & Zondervan
1663 Liberty Drive
Bloomington, IN 47403
www.westbowpress.com
1 (866) 928-1240

Because of the dynamic nature of the Internet, any web addresses or
links contained in this book may have changed since publication and
may no longer be valid. The views expressed in this work are solely those
of the author and do not necessarily reflect the views of the publisher,
and the publisher hereby disclaims any responsibility for them.

Any people depicted in stock imagery provided by Thinkstock are models,
and such images are being used for illustrative purposes only.
Certain stock imagery © Thinkstock.

ISBN: 978-1-5127-8002-4 (sc)
ISBN: 978-1-5127-8003-1 (hc)
ISBN: 978-1-5127-8004-8 (e)

Library of Congress Control Number: 2017904255

Print information available on the last page.

WestBow Press rev. date: 12/07/2017

Table of Contents

Table of Contents

Endorsement

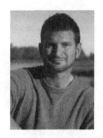

Brad Bloom,
Publisher, Faith and Fitness Magazine

Finding a straightforward resource to help you improve your physical activity can be difficult. That's why I really like Donald Steven's book *METAMORFIT – 21 Day Journey To A Better You.* His book is easy to read and simple to use. The daily exercises don't require equipment and can be done anywhere whenever you want to take a short break during your day. Like many faith-based fitness books he includes daily prayers. Nice? Yes! But, he doesn't stop there. Donald shares faith insights that challenge you to pursue greater strength in God. That's what makes this much more than the usual fitness guide. His spirited faith-centered message is strategic to help you pursue the transformation God has for you.

-Brad Bloom, Publisher,
Faith & Fitness Magazine, faithandfitness.net

Preface

God is doing something great in the world today. When that greatness is revealed to each person a change in form and habits occur. It's a physical and spiritual metamorphosis. It's the ultimate in getting and staying fit.

Bobby was a pot smoker looking for something more. He wasn't satisfied. His childhood was scary, his family life was conflicted and his personal life had been traumatic. When I met Bobby he was sixteen and hanging out with the wrong crowd. He was spiritually hurting. His physical body was hurting too. As he observed my active lifestyle he wanted to know how he could have the same kind of strength, energy and joy. God places people like Bobby around us all the time. To open our eyes to them and respond with grace and hope is to release the greatness of God. When I yielded to God to be used in Bobby's life, he was forever changed.

There's a lot going on in our world today. We're moving and motivated by what we see and feel. For Bobby, my fitness then my faith influenced him to find God. However, there are many influences that can take us far from who we are created to be – our greater potential and purpose. I see people distracted and consumed by the chaos in their lives. As a personal trainer, I'm a missionary. My mission is to help people depart from the chaos, achieve change, and experience the power and might of God.

Historically, we know that thousands of missionaries have traveled to nations preaching the gospel of Jesus Christ, healing the sick, and giving to the needy. Poor physical health and wellness can be a key factor in slowing their ministry work or bringing it to a complete stop. I'm not talking about health and wellness as it relates to age. There is a natural process for older evangelists and missionaries to mentor and then hand off the torch to a successor to continue the work.

Those that get ill due to carelessness, a lack of eating healthy or maintaining proper exercise, defeat their purpose and often fail to see the fullness of their potential. Do we blame the devil for such a loss or should they take responsibility for their own neglect?

Both play a role. But – shift your focus now from the many distant missionaries throughout the world to you. Today in your part of the world you can be a missionary. Don't make a distinction between 'them' and 'you'. Everyone can make a positive impact in the lives of others. Moreover, those who identify as Christian have a clear calling and time-tested instruction (the Bible) to do it well. Sure, evil abounds to kill, steel and destroy. So, don't be defenseless.

This twenty-one day devotional is designed to help you do daily physical and spiritual exercise so you can maintain a healthy and fit lifestyle and remain on your missionary field for as long as possible. These exercises are critically important for you to be fit to do the good work of helping others. Taking care of your body means doing your part to be faithful in the processes of daily health and miraculous healing.

This book is a tool for everyone. I believe it will cause you to ask questions and research the Bible. This guide can help you make better fitness and spiritual choices. It can give you a new perspective – a solid mindset of how health and fitness is a lifestyle rather than a short-term diet. I pray that this book will empower you in many ways, cause you to value Christ's instruction and mature the way you think about your spirit, soul, and body.

Laying the Foundation
Spirit, Soul, and Body

May God, who makes everything holy and whole, make YOU holy and whole, created and structured together spirit, soul, and body and keep you fit for the coming of our Lord, Jesus Christ.

1 Thessalonians 5:23

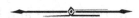

From the very foundations of the earth human civilization has been built. Though we journey one generation to the next from birth, through life to death, we continue to wonder at the great mysteries of our origin. We know from reading the Book of Genesis that the creation of earth and heaven by God was a supernatural event that is beyond human understanding. To accept and celebrate God's handiwork requires faith. It's by faith that we can comprehend the creation of God by his word and his invisible presence. This is important to understand as you lay a foundation for a stronger approach to your physical fitness. God created all things physical and they are a direct reflection of His spiritual nature.

Beyond God speaking the world into existence He also created male and female to take care of His creation. Genesis 2:7 (MSG) says, **GOD formed Man out of dirt from the ground and blew into his nostrils the breath of life. The Man came alive—a living soul!**, Three things happen in this one Bible verse.

First, God formed man out of the dust of the ground. Dust by itself can't take form. Water is needed to shape and mold it. Genesis 2:5-6 (MSG) says, "**At the time GOD made Earth and Heaven, before any grasses or shrubs had sprouted from the ground—GOD hadn't yet sent rain on Earth, nor was there anyone around to work the ground (the whole Earth was watered by underground springs)**". God in His creative ability took the mud and created a man with every detail in His body with the ability to work in His Garden. God gave man the tools He knew was necessary to make sure that God's creation was well taken care of.

Second, God breathed into man's nostrils the breath of life. God designed us to physically receive His image and likeness. The Word breath in Hebrew is *ruach* (roo-akh), which means spirit. Man was given a spirit so that he can stay connected with God. God created man from His own image and likeness, and God is a Spirit which means that our body contains the image of God. The existence of God can't be seen with natural eyes because He is a spirit and the only way to serve and worship God is in spirit and the understanding of the truth of His word. However, our spirits became tainted – separated from that true worship and fellowship with God- after the fall of man (the willful act of disobedience and sinfulness). Through Jesus we have restoration. Through the Holy Spirit, which is the Spirit of God, we can stay connected with Him as originally designed.

Third, man became a living soul after God gave him life. Without the spirit the soul and body are dead. James 2:26 tells us that without the spirit our body is dead. I will go into greater detail about the soul later. For now, let's simply discuss that man was created in the following three parts: spirit, soul and body. Paul in the New Testament speaks to all of us when he says that God wants our whole body (spirit, soul, and body) to be preserved unto Christ. Before willful sin, humanity was perfect following God's plan to till the garden and have dominion over the earth. Without

Christ's redemption that sin nature makes it impossible for us to stay connected to God and treat our body the way God sees it — perfect.

The Body

—————➤●◀—————

Our body was created specifically to glorify God not ourselves. We're the vessels in which God lives. He displays His love through us and shines His light so the world may know Him. God doesn't dwell in a building made with hands. Did you know that your body is the actual house or temple of God? Many people today would answer that question with a "No". They don't know that we're created to host the Holy Spirit so that God's perfect will can be done. It is hard to believe that a supreme God would dwell in such imperfect vessels like ours.

Jesus Christ came to earth to reveal the heart of God and to show us that there is a better way. Jesus prayed that we would be one with God just as He was one with Him. The only way for us to be one with God is through the blood of Jesus Christ. It was through His sacrifice and the giving of His Spirit that we are made right with God. God's presence is like pure treasure, and we are the vessels that carry the treasure. His love and grace has nothing to do with our ability but with who he is.

We need to recognize that our body not just our spirit is to be kept honorable and blameless. Most people agree that their body isn't meant for evil — to be a weapon or sex object. But, too few realize they were created to bring glory to God just as Jesus did.

They don't recognize that there is a spiritual realm. If they do they often segregate it to some nominal religious ritual that has little bearing on life. Our natural body has five senses: taste, touch, smell, hearing, and sight. These five senses give us the ability to interact with the natural world around us. If you were pinched in the arm you would automatically respond to the feeling. If you smelled a delicious apple pie your mouth would probably begin to water even before you taste it.

Our bodies are so familiar with the physical realm that we involuntarily respond – it's automatic. If we would behave with the understanding that our body is the window to our spirit, our spiritual response can also become involuntary and automatic. That is why it is important to take care of our bodies. Eating right and exercising vigorously are both physical and spiritual practices. 1 Timothy 4:8 (AMP) says, **"For physical training is of some value, but godliness (spiritual training) is of value in everything *and* in every way, since it holds promise for the present life and for the life to come."**

Paul's comparison of bodily exercise alongside godliness (exercising the spirit) is dramatic because physical gains are temporary while spiritual gains last forever. But that doesn't mean physical fitness has no value. Many people, especially Christians, twist this Bible passage to justify not working out and staying in shape. Much research has been done and evidence abounds that physical exercise results in a stronger and healthier body and yields many 'spiritual' benefits too.

Science aside, the men and women in the Bible were probably some of the fittest people on earth. They didn't struggle with the temptation of fast food restaurants and processed foods you can heat in the microwave. It's also unlikely that their bodies hurt from being too sedentary. However, they also didn't have access to a gym the way we do, especially when we feel convicted after eating heavy on holidays. Most of their time were spent walking long distances to different cities to buy food, and tools for shelter.

Jesus may not have been the biggest guy in the world, but He sure was fit. As a Rabbi (a Jewish scholar or teacher) He maintained a strict diet according to Jewish laws. He also walked extensively and often climbed a mountain to spend time in prayer. As a result of His spiritual exercise, I suspect Jesus developed strong, powerful legs. His disciples apparently didn't have as much stamina – the Bible notes they couldn't stay awake while he prayed. Christ's consistent physical training ultimately had a very physical role in his most pivotal spiritual act. He carried His cross, four times His weight, was crucified and gave His life for all humanity. His focus was automatically and continually on doing God's will not on being in shape physically. Yet, without question the greater could not have been done without the lesser. That is the example we all must follow.

The Spirit

Many people don't understand the things of God. They believe that to be led by God's spirit is to lose control. It is counter to their daily existence and sinful nature. Therefore, Christians need to take serious their role in demonstrating spiritual living. By doing that it makes spiritual concepts more tangible. The spirit of God is released in the lives of others when Christians demonstrate the power of God daily. It is through this power that people can start to come alive to truthful living and be less sucked in by lies.

These days it can be difficult to know what is real and what is fake. Once reputable news sources now have credibility issues. Photos and videos can now be manipulated to alter our perception of reality. Additives to the foods we eat not only call into question the accuracy of the labeling but leaves us to raise concerns about their impact on our bodies. We've come to realize that our confidence in the tangible and physical as reality is not certain. The reality is more often built on our best knowledge and our hope for something reliable.

At the same time, while Bible truths will always require faith, the spirit of God produces fruit in the lives of people – tangible positive results that release a non-tangible power. Spiritual living connects you to something you may not fully understand, but it's a greater strength you can certainly feel.

God, in the beginning, spoke this natural world into being. Without the spiritual realm the natural realm doesn't exist. This is a key understanding. It helps you to shift from the traditional concepts of being fit to being metamorfit. It is the spirit, not the body that is in control.

The Soul

———▶●◀———

Our soul is a very important part of who we are as humans. The soul contains our mind, emotions, desires and consciousness. Sometimes people say they feel the presence of God in church, but what is actually happening is that their soul which contains emotions is responding to the living Spirit of God in them. Our body can sometimes respond to what our soul is feeling which is giving us a sense of God's presence.

Our soul is like a pipeline for the Spirit of God to move through. But just like any pipe, it must be clean so that you get the pure spirit of God rather than a compromise. The valve on our soul also must be open so that the fruit of the Spirit can flow as well. If we keep our soul dirty and closed to the Spirit, then our body, our spirit and those around us will never fully be able to reap the benefits of God.

It is important to understand how your soul can be led by God's spirit. We identify some people as angry or tortured souls. Whether you believe in Satan or not, they seem to be led by darkness, hate, despair, anger, sadness --- everything that is destructive to them and those around them. Other people are much more positive, but they only self-feed and strengthen their soul. They educate their mind, try to keep emotionally positive, struggle to have pure desires and try to demonstrate some reasonable awareness of others. These good works are only as strong as the limits of their human capacity.

It is only when the soul is led by God's spirit that we can love those who show us hate. The soul led by God's spirit can persevere when there is no logical hope. A spirit-led soul can have the purity of heart to desire only the will of God. A good soul is not a bad soul, but it does deny the spirit of God. In contrast, the soul fixed on God transcends the limits of our physical world and taps into the limitless potential of God's spirit.

A tortured soul lives for himself or herself only, "I need to look out for me only."

A good soul donates to a worthy cause and then gets on with life.

A soul led by God's spirit is ready to be inconvenienced and looks for ways to use its strengths for the unique benefit of an individual in need. This is what it means to be metamorFit.

MetamorFit

Do not be conformed to this world, but be transformed by the renewal of your mind, that by testing you may discern what is the will of God, what is good and acceptable and perfect.

Romans 12:2

Throughout the United States Klove radio and both *The Message* and *Kirk Franklin's Praise* on Sirius XM satellite radio are a continuous source of Christian music for millions of listeners. Most people today can't remember a time when Contemporary Christian Music wasn't an industry within itself and readily accessible. It's a genre that started in the late 60's during a cultural revolution known as the Jesus Movement. Before that there were basically just hymns. The style gave musicians the ability to do what Jesus had done centuries earlier – share faith in a simple and relatable way. It transformed how people, young and old, experience Christianity. In 1978 a Barry McGuire children's recording related the concept of being "born again" to the metamorphosis of *Bullfrogs and Butterflies*. In much the same way, I've written this book because I believe it can help you make clear connections between a fit lifestyle and the Christian faith.

According to Strong's Concordance, the Greek word for 'transformed' is metamorphoo (Strong's Concordance, p. 3339), which is where we get the English word "metamorphosis." The word meta (Strong's Concordance, p. 3326), means "change after being with" and morphoo (Stong's Concordance, p. 3445), means "changing form in keeping with inner reality." In the Bible Paul teaches that we should present our bodies a living sacrifice, holy, acceptable unto God. Transformation doesn't instantly happen when you accept the saving grace of Christ; it is a process. Our mind is renewed as we deny ourselves and submit to God.

We mature with time physically and spiritually. Think about what that looks like for you. A few of us seem to age gracefully and are told that the years have been good to us. Most settle for something less flattering and perhaps even hopeless, "Life sucks and then you die." The world in which we live is an ever-present force as we mature. Jesus experienced humanity to share that in common with us. Paul encourages us not to conform to this world, but he wasn't speaking about the outer man. He was talking about the inner man. Change begins in the inner man before it takes shape in the outer man. That is the basis for Metamorfit.

What is Metamorfit?

I created the term 'Metamorfit' after investing a full year in trying to understand who I am in Christ. I felt an urgency to find my identity as a child of God. I listened in prayer, and He began to speak to me about my diet and about the importance of being fit to do the work of the ministry. I wasn't chubby, but I knew I needed to lose weight and get leaner.

I gradually started replacing certain foods like pork, beef, and chicken with more vegetables and eventually became a part-time vegan. This lifestyle forced me to work out much harder because I wasn't getting the amount of protein I needed to gain lean muscles. During the two-months diet I lost over thirty pounds and gained muscle. But – I gained something greater. I learned how to daily live life faithfully for God. My thinking was transformed with God's perspective rather than a secular worldview. I felt more confident, not in myself but in Christ. Each day I made it my mission to encourage others to pursue a different kind of fitness. A fitness not after the flesh but after the Spirit so they too could do God's work.

To be 'metamorfit' is to be aware of who you are, whose you are, and to live transformed by the renewing of your mind according to God's instruction. It also means to live with an awareness of your body in the context of taking care of what God created. Metamorfit focuses on the inner man as well as the outer man through exercising both spirit and body.

On the other hand, some secular programs like yoga call for you to empty yourself and be one with nature. Some poses can also include worshipping idols. God desires us to be one with Him. MetamorFit helps you look to Him for answers not to yourself. Although yoga has physical benefits, spiritually it doesn't connect you with God and His words in the Bible.

For the next twenty-one days use this book to daily meditate on Bible passages that will focus on the spirit and the soul. The book provides you with encouraging daily words and a prayer followed by a daily workout routine. This isn't a Bible study (though I hope it makes you want to study your Bible more). It is a guide to support you through the day with a greater awareness of God's Spirit. It can help you respond to different daily situations using the Fruit of the Spirit. It is designed to help you become more health conscious, more aware of your body, and do something maybe you've never done before --- treat it with reverence (deep respect regarding it as valuable to God).

I've also created space for you to journal what God speaks to you after reading the selected Bible verse and throughout the day. Of course you need to actively listen to hear that. Journal how you felt after the workout and what you eat daily. Combining physical and faith insights will help you stay on top of your health and spiritual goals. The daily prayer is just a simple start. It gives you a foundation on which I want you to build a more robust personal prayer time with God. Reflect on the Bible verse as you pray. Become aware of God's Spirit in you and anticipate God revealing to you new insights about you.

The workout routines can be done anytime during the day. I really encourage you to try and do all the workouts. This helps you build discipline, do things that may be out of your comfort zone and begin your transformation in Christ.

Nutrition

I'm not a nutritionist. However, eating healthy and clean food will benefit you in so many ways. My website www.iammetamorfit.com provides a variety of nutrition references and resources. When God created the earth He created it with foods that He engineered to keep us healthy and live a strong life. Furthermore, God gave us his creative nature to combine these foods with flavorful herbs and cooking techniques and make meals that celebrate the goodness of God. Many commercially produced foods are a far cry from what God intended for us.

Like Daniel and the three Hebrew boys in the Bible you can choose to eat right. What is right? Be wise, do research, pray and seek God and then make food choices that will be healthier for you. You'll find that eating the right food and drinking water will increase clarity of the mind, increase energy, clear up the skin and give you many other benefits.

I have experienced all of the above, and I have committed to healthy eating as a lifestyle rather than a diet. To repent means to simply change your mind or your way of thinking. Christians today often use the word "repent" to encourage or sometimes attempt to force others to turn to Christ and turn away from sinful ways. That's not how it works. Repentance isn't just turning away from sin. It also requires a change in thinking from a soul that does good to a soul that is spirit-led. What if you repent from the way you eat and turn to healthy eating? What if you repent from the way you think about how you look and instead work out daily ? Those are good things to do, but they won't truly be transformative until you are led by God's spirit. When you do that what will YOU look like?

There is a better YOU compared to how you see yourself right now. There is a way that God sees you right now, but if you don't change your way of thinking when it comes to nutrition, fitness, and spiritual growth, your better YOU will always be hidden from those around you. They are waiting to see the better YOU.

This journey may be tough for you. I believe when you finish these twenty-one days that you will feel more confident in who you are in God. These daily exercises for your body and daily readings for your spirit will give you a different perspective of yourself and others. God help us pursue a transformation of body, soul and spirit.

Let's Get Metamorfit!

Before Your Journey

1.: Go to www.iammetamorfit.com
2.: Click the Login/Sign up button on the right hand side

LOGIN/SIGN UP

3.: Sign up using your Facebook, or Email account
4.: In the Guest Area type in the password: metamorfitlife

Note:

The exercises selected for this book provide you with a means to be active and physically experience being metamorfit. Some movements may require jumping and the bending of the knees. Consult your Doctor to discuss your abilities, limitations and any recommended precautions before performing these moves, especially if you have health issues or are pregnant. The exercises can be modified as needed. You'll find ideas to adapt the exercises on my website.

For information on nutrition and healthy eating, please visit:

www.iammetamorfit.com/nutrition

Day 1

What's on your Mind?

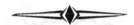

*I Am No Longer Bound to the
law of sin and death
I Am free in Christ Jesus*
Romans 8:2

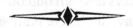

What's on your Mind?

If you live to only please the flesh, your mind will only be set on what the flesh needs; but if you live according to the Spirit, then your mind will set on what the Spirit desires. The mind that is driven by the flesh will result in an unexpected end, but the mind that is driven by the Spirit is life and peace.

Romans 8:5-6

The famous Facebook status question, "What's on your mind" was introduced so users can express how they are feeling in that moment. It may be tough to admit but not every thought we entertain is a good one. Someone might cut us off on the highway so we give them an angry look and reciprocate with rudeness. Perhaps the waiter might have messed up our order so we may have a few choice words to say that are hurtful and bring discouragement. What we think and what we say will always have an outcome producing either good fruit or bad fruit. We have a choice. Paul says that to be carnally minded (to have worldly passions) is death. You negatively affect the lives of others, often in ways you can't even realize, when your attitude is self-driven and your approach to life lacks commitment to values. Instead, we are encouraged to seek after God's mindset and wisdom so that in all of life, not just when situations arise, we can anticipate that God will shape the outcome. Jesus Christ makes this possible. This is true not just for when we're around others but also for when we are alone. It's said that eighty percent of the time our voice is the only thing we believe. Our angry words and negative thoughts hurt our own spirit and damage our bodies. When we speak and live according to God's words, we will walk in His life. I encourage you to speak life according to God's word. So, what's on your mind today?

Prayer

Father, I thank You that through Christ, who is seated at Your right hand, we have access to everything that is pure and holy. Father, forgive me for entertaining the thoughts that come to my mind that does not edify You. Show me what I must seek according to Your Word so that every word that I speak will become fruitful and multiply to those around me. Father, I thank You that I am created in Your image and likeness and that this body that You have formed is healthy. Thank You for Your Word that gives life.

Exercise: Day 1

Movement	Sets	Repetitions	Rest
Jumping-Jacks	4	20	15sec
Crunches	4	20	15sec
Push-ups	4	10-20	1 minute than repeat

Each workout should be done in order with the given amount of rest in between. After the first set of each movement, rest for 1 minute and repeat the cycle of exercise movements. If you want to challenge yourself do more repetitions.

Visit https://www.iammetamorfit.com/21-day-journey for workouts

Journal Your Day

_____
_____
_____
_____
_____
_____
_____
_____
_____
_____
_____
_____
_____
_____
_____
_____
_____
_____
_____
_____
_____
_____
_____
_____
_____
_____
_____
_____
_____
_____
_____

Day 2

God's Free Gift

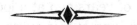

I Am delivered from the power of darkness and translated into the kingdom of light of Jesus Christ
Colossians 1:13

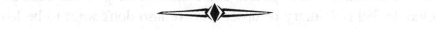

God's Free Gift

We haven't received spirit of this world, but the Spirit who came from God. This happened so that we might know and understand the things freely given to us by God.

1 Corinthians 2:12

I met Yolanda a couple of years ago at a local juice and smoothie shop. Most everyone working at this energy-infused store seemed to have a good time mixing healthy fresh flavors --- except Yolanda. More often than not she always had a sad countenance. When I asked her how she was doing her answer was the typical, "Oh I'm fine." But her facial expression told a whole other story.

Maybe you identify with her and put up a front so that nobody can see how horrible you feel on the inside. Our body has a job, and that job is to animate what is spiritual according to God's Word or to animate our feelings and emotions according to our soul. It's okay to feel sad, angry or upset; but we also don't want to be led by those emotions daily. God has given us His Spirit that we may know the things which are freely given by Him. And those things are true, honest, pure, lovely, and of good report. So, when we think about these things daily our countenance will always be joyous and exciting. However, not everyone thinks on these things daily, maybe not even often or at all. You can make a difference.

Christians, led by God's Spirit, can live a more vibrant, joyous and purposeful life as the Bible promises and instructs. Not every day may be a happy juice day, but we should animate the heart of God and put aside our own feelings so that God can lift us above our frustrations and darkness. We can then help others. I committed to do that with Yolanda. Instead of just hoping she'd see Jesus in me, I actively searched for opportunities that God created for me to extend His grace to her. Over time she too came to find the joy and peace of God's free gift.

Prayer

Father, show me what is true, honest, pure, lovely, and of good report so that I can express Your heart and desire to others. I don't want to be led by my emotions but by Your Spirit which You have given to me freely. Father, I thank You that You have given me a better way and that way is through Jesus. God, help me to appreciate You even when things don't seem right. I know that as I do, Your Word will back up my praise. Thank You for Your joy, Your comfort and for guiding g me through Your Word.

Exercise: Day 2

Movement	Sets	Repetitions	Rest
Mountain Climbers	4	15	15
Pushups	4	5-20	15
Reverse Crunch	4	10-20	15
Planks	4	30sec-1minute	1minute than repeat

Each workout should be done in order with the given amount of rest in between. After the first set of each movement, rest for 1 minute and repeat the cycle of exercise movements. If you want to challenge yourself do more repetitions.

Visit https://www.iammetamorfit.com/21-day-journey for workouts

_____

_____

_____

_____

_____

_____

_____

_____

_____

_____

_____

_____

_____

_____

_____

_____

_____

_____

_____

_____

_____

_____

_____

_____

_____

_____

_____

_____

_____

_____

_____

_____

_____

_____

Day 3

Holy Spirit Our Helper

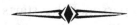

I Am not the same person anymore
I Am a new creation in Christ
2 Corinthians 5:17

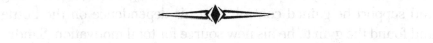

Holy Spirit Our Helper

Prepare your mind, stay alert, and stay hopeful on the grace that was given to you for the return of our Lord, Jesus Christ

1 Peter 1:13

Someone that may have had too much to drink is unstable in his mind and body. This may cause embarrassment to him or herself and to those around that person. What starts happening is that their mind and body will lose all control, and the chemical that they put in their body will now take over. The word "gird" simply means to bind. When something is bound you have control over it.

Sandra and Dwayne were one of many couples in Detroit impacted by industry changes and a bad economy. Dwayne hadn't just lost his job, he'd lost hope too. That loss led to depression, alcohol addiction, inactivity and weight gain. Eventually, through counseling and support he gained control, beat his dependence on the bottle and found the gym to be his new source for total motivation. Sandra prayed for something more – and God delivered. Dwayne discovered that even his best intentions and accomplishments needed to be given to God to achieve true strength and a redeemed identity.

Having a sober mind means to have a clear and stable mind. It means having control of your own thoughts and actions. But God wants to take it a step further. If we control our mind then there is no room for the mind of Christ. He wants us to see that the way we are thinking may not be the best way. We should gird up that part of our mind so that we can bring our body into subjection. Our body will only do what our mind entertains for a long period of time. Chances are that if we think about something for a while we will become doers of our thoughts. But God wants us to be a doer of His word and not become a castaway. The Holy Spirit as our helper is there to guide us into all truth. He is there to help us in our weak areas through intercession. It's a great feeling to know that even if we don't have the right words to say, the Holy Spirit searches our hearts and makes intercession on our behalf according to God's will.

Prayers

Father, I acknowledge that the Holy Spirit is my helper, and He is making intercession for me according to Your word. Father, as I go through the day, I will encounter things and situations that may be out of my control. I know though that You are my peace, and You will guide me into all truth. Father, forgive me if I have indulged in my own thoughts and became drunk, losing control of my true identity in You. Help me bring my mind and my body back into subjection according to Your will and purpose.

Exercise: Day 3 (***recovery day if you choose to**)

Movement	Sets	Repetitions	Rest
Running place	4	15-30	15sec
Jumping Jacks	4	15-30	15sec
Mountain Climbers	4	10-20	1 minute that repeat

*Each workout should be done in order with the given amount of rest in between. After the first set of each movement, rest for 1 minute and repeat the cycle of exercise movements. If you want to challenge yourself do more repetitions.

Visit https://www.iammetamorfit.com/21-day-journey for workouts

Journal Your Day

Day 4

I Have Love, Power, and a Sound Mind

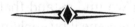

I Am God's wonderful creation in Christ Jesus
I Am ordained to walk in good works
Ephesians 2:10

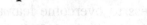

I Have Love, Power, and a Sound Mind

**For God gave us a spirit not of fear but of
power and love and self-control.**

2 Timothy 1:7 (ESV)

Fear is the biggest obstacle that will prevent us from moving forward into the purpose that God has for us. Fear has been a stumbling block for many people. When we understand that fear is not something that God gives we can overcome it by applying the truth of the Bible. Our mind becomes sound when we set it on things above.

Tanji Johnson is a well-respected fitness coach, former Air Force officer and six-time IFBB Pro Fitness title holder. Through her successful fitness business she coaches women internationally always with a high commitment to ministering God's grace and love. It took a lot of hard work to get to where she is today. It took prayer and a willingness to overcome fear and to be vulnerable. Tanji says, "Vulnerability is all about feeling exposed to emotional hurt. We've all been there and it is not fun. Often we are left feeling weak and fragile and susceptible of being taken advantage of. The thought of relating your innermost feelings and fears to someone with the possibility of them not caring or even using them against you is straight up SCARY!"

When we allow our mind to fear rather than trust God we are slowly extinguishing or quenching the Spirit. When something is quenched, it can no longer be in use. God has given us His Spirit through His Son, Jesus Christ, so that He can help us. If we quench the Spirit we are led to fear things that we shouldn't. Fear allowed to persist can lead to sin which can affect our body.

Tanji has learned how to overcome fear. She explains, "I am joyful to be able to proclaim the freedom of true vulnerability! I know that deep in our core, God made us to need each other in addition to Him so that we can experience new possibilities, receive help, develop trust in others… be in tune with our real feelings and let go of fears."

To be MetamorFit is to trust in God, be filled with His power and love and have a sound mind. We are free from sin and fear through Jesus Christ.

Prayer

Father, I thank You that you have given me love, power, and sound mind through Your Spirit. I no longer fear what comes my way. Forgive me, Lord, if I have slipped back into my carnal mind and ways because of fear. Forgive me, Lord, if I have quenched the Spirit for my own self-gain. I thank You, Father, that You have given me Your Word to guide me and Your Spirit to help me. Lord, teach me what it means to have a sound mind and not be led by any fear that comes.

Exercise: Day 4

Movement	Sets	Repetitions	Rest
Running in Place	4	10-20	15sec
Front Squats	4	10-15	15sec

| Single leg Lunges | 4 | 10-15 | 15sec |
| Jumping Jacks | 4 | 10-15 | 1 minute than repeat |

Each workout should be done in order with the given amount of rest in between. After the first set of each movement, rest for 1 minute and repeat the cycle of exercise movements. If you want to challenge yourself do more repetitions.

Visit https://www.iammetamorfit.com/21-day-journey for workouts

Journal Your Day

Day 5

I am in the Spirit

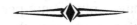

I Am a representative of Christ
I Am reconciled to God

2 Corinthians 5:20

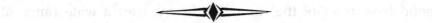

I am in the Spirit

You, however, are not in the flesh but in the Spirit, if in fact the Spirit of God dwells in you. Anyone who does not have the Spirit of Christ does not belong to him.

Romans 8:9 (ESV)

I was told we act selfishly eighty percent of the time and the way God would have us behave only twenty percent of the time. Why the disparity? Perhaps it's because even though we say we want to get fit and strong, we don't want to do the work to make it happen. It's easy to remain as an infant and want to please our flesh. We cry when we're hungry, cry when we're tired, and cry when we want to be picked up.

Jamel is one of the most interesting guys you'll ever find at the gym. At first glance he seems to be doing a lot right. He has good form most of the time, lifts heavy, uses a wide range of supplements and muscle builders and hits the gym every day for over an hour. So, you may wonder why he's not a cover model material. He's not actually in all that great of shape. Turns out he has cheat meal regularly. His commitment to family, work and God isn't near as regular as his gym time. When things don't go well – watch out for that temper. In the spirit and the flesh he represents immaturity.

As children we act out our desires with emotions so that we can get what we want. As we get older as teenagers and adults, this selfish way of life can go on for years. This mindset is opposed and in fact hostile to God. It is a stubbornness that keeps us from achieving change and being able to mature and do God's will. We claim to have the Spirit of Christ but we still live by the flesh.

If we have the Spirit of God in us He will quickly reroute our way of thinking about what is acceptable to Him. We renew our mind by realizing that the way we are thinking is not the will of God. This renewed mind enables us to be coachable, attentive to His voice and to be trained daily in the Bible. As we do this our actions will reflect His true strength. We will be in the Spirit and reconciled to God with a strength that is truly representative of Christ.

Prayer

Father, I thank You that you have given me the same Spirit that raised up Jesus Christ from the dead. It is by that same Spirit that we can walk according to Your perfect will for us. Father, I confess that I have been living according to the flesh and not by the Spirit which You gave to me. I pray that You would teach me how to walk according to the Spirit and not the flesh. I no longer want to be conformed to the world's way of thinking; I want to be transformed by the renewing of my mind to the mind of Christ which was given through salvation by faith. Teach me Your ways, Lord, so that I can continue to live in Your perfect will for me.

Exercise: Day 5

Movement	Sets	Repetitions	Rest
Mountain Climbers	3	10-20	15sec
Push-ups	3	5-20	15sec
Planks	3	20sec-1minute	1minute than repeat

Each workout should be done in order with the given amount of rest in between. After the first set of each movement, rest for 1 minute and repeat the cycle of exercise movements. If you want to challenge yourself do more repetitions.

Visit https://www.iammetamorfit.com/21-day-journey for workouts

Journal Your Day

_____
_____
_____
_____
_____
_____
_____
_____
_____
_____
_____
_____
_____
_____
_____
_____
_____
_____
_____
_____
_____
_____
_____
_____
_____
_____
_____
_____

Day 6

Am I walking in the Spirit?

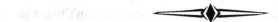

I Am a light of this world
Matthew 5:14

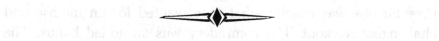

Am I walking in the Spirit?

**If you walk in the Spirit, then you will
not manifest the lust of the flesh.**

Galatians 5:16

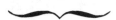

Have you ever heard the expression that you are your own worst enemy? Well, that can be very true in most cases. Our worldly saturated minds fight against our spirit and against God. The Bible talks quite a bit about the struggle within. Satan doesn't want us to have any part of God's will and desire. Internally the evil one tries to persuade you to go a different way and alienate you from a loving God. The battle is constant and the only way to win on a day-to-day basis is to understand first that the battle is God's.

Erik and Janice were a young couple who found their local CrossFit box was exactly what they wanted for an intense and challenging workout. The comradery was an added bonus. The extra accountability pushed them to make amazing gains. It also led quite unexpectedly to an invitation to a regular gathering of members to talk about faith, which they accepted. Before long they were being challenged in a very different way. Confronting lustful desires for social and financial gain, arrogance and dishonesty gave them a workout that was more challenging than any WOD (Workout of The Day).

Begin today to walk in the Spirit according to what you learn in the Bible and through the good example and support of others. When you do that you'll find strength from God to better resist the things that battle within your mind. You'll forge a greater strength to be metamorfit. Your body is the vessel to celebrate God's Spirit. He has won the battle for us on the cross.

Prayer

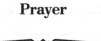

Father, I thank You for sending Your son Jesus to win this battle that I am currently fighting in my mind. I thank You, Father, that I am a new creation through Jesus Christ, and I no longer live by my carnal feelings but by the Holy Spirit. Father, as I walk after the Spirit direct me and show me how to maintain a steady balance in the Word so that I will not stumble and fall into the flesh. My desire is to please You. Help me follow Your Word and Your teachings.

Exercise: Day 6

Movement	Sets	Repetitions	Rest
Running in place	4	15-20	15sec
Leg raises	4	10-20	15sec
Crunches	4	10-20	45 sec than repeat

Each workout should be done in order with the given amount of rest in between. After the first set of each movement, rest for 1 minute and repeat the cycle of exercise movements. If you want to challenge yourself do more repetitions.

Visit https://www.iammetamorfit.com/21-day-journey for workouts

Journal Your Day

_____

_____

_____

_____

_____

_____

_____

_____

_____

_____

_____

_____

_____

_____

_____

_____

_____

_____

_____

_____

_____

_____

_____

_____

_____

_____

_____

Day 7

Where does your Peace come from?

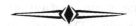

I Am built up in Christ Jesus
I Am rooted in Christ Jesus
I Am established in my faith in Christ Jesus
Colossians 2:6-7

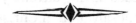

Where does your Peace come from?

**You keep him in perfect peace whose mind is
stayed on you because he trusts in you.**

Isaiah 26:3

It's amazing how the world views peace today. Ending world hunger, putting an end to war and violence, everyone coming together as one no matter what race, gender orientation, religion, or political views are just a few examples. This may all seem great and sounds hopeful to many that form movements and different clubs. But the fact of the matter is there is only one true God that can you give you perfect peace. This peace is not external but internal.

Briant K. Mitchell owns BKM Fitness Boot Camp in Ferguson, Missouri. When unrest broke out in 2014, businesses all around him were destroyed. He knew God's blessing was upon him with only two broken windows, and he never closed. His faith in God gave him tremendous peace during adversity and joy that continues to draw people. For Briant salvation in Christ is so much more than just having hope to survive until eternity. It is renewing his mind, reshaping his body and helping others all around him do the same.

This is a peace that passes all understanding of the carnal view of peace. Isaiah says that if we keep our mind on God then we will have that peace, and I believe it will remain forever. We were given the helmet of salvation which is Jesus and the sword of the Spirit which is also Jesus. Perfect peace only comes from Jesus Christ, and it is given freely if you accept it. He doesn't want us to have a troubled heart or be afraid. Jesus didn't just die so that we can get into heaven. He died so that we can establish right standing and a relationship with our Father. Jesus came so that He might be manifest in our mortal flesh. Now His peace and His Word can live with us forever.

Prayer

Father, I thank You that you sent your son Jesus Christ to die not only for me to make it into heaven, but also to have eternal peace here on earth. Father, forgive me for not acknowledging that You are peace and that the world can't offer me peace. You have given me your Word and salvation, and now I have peace with You. Lord, help me to walk in the peace that I have already through Your Son, Jesus Christ, and don't ever let Your words depart from me. Father, I thank You that Jesus now takes residence in my mortal flesh so that I don't live by bread alone but by every word that proceeded out of Your mouth.

Exercise: Day 7 (***recovery day if you choose to**)

Movement	Sets	Repetitions	Rest
Mountain Climbers	3	10-15	15sec
Running in Place	3	10-15	15sec
Jumping Jacks	3	10-15	1minute than repeat

Each workout should be done in order with the given amount of rest in between. After the first set of each movement, rest for 1 minute and repeat the cycle of exercise movements. If you want to challenge yourself do more repetitions.

_____

_____

_____

_____

_____

_____

_____

_____

_____

_____

_____

_____

_____

_____

_____

_____

_____

_____

_____

_____

_____

_____

_____

_____

_____

_____

_____

_____

Day 8

God's words of Life

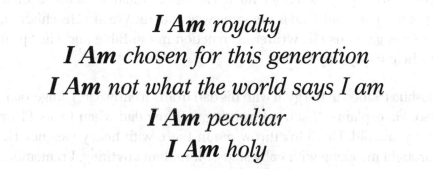

I Am royalty
I Am chosen for this generation
I Am not what the world says I am
I Am peculiar
I Am holy

God's words of Life

Jesus answered, "It is written: 'Man shall not live on bread alone, but on every word that comes from the mouth of God.

Matthew 4:4 (NIV)

A father will always know what is best for his children. He will create rules and provide leadership not to annoy them but to simply make sure they don't get hurt. He wants them to achieve their greatest potential. God is the same way with us. We are His children. He has given us His written instruction in the Bible and His Spirit to help us joyfully follow.

Joshua trained in the gym with his dad from an early age. Dangerous? No. He explains, "I started training with my dad when I was 11 or 12 years old. He didn't throw me in there with heavy weights. He brought me along with baby steps. More than anything, I remember he wanted me to get the technique." Today, Joshua Haney's Facebook profile reads: Son of the Most High God, 1st Lt. of my father 8-time Mr. Olympia, Lee Haney. He is the Chief Operating Officer of Lee Haney Nutrition among many other things.

God brings instructions back to our remembrance if we fall of course. Sometimes, we fall into the temptation of allowing worldly desires to fill our hearts. Howver, we have an advocate, and when we ask for forgiveness we know that we will have another chance to be in right standing with God. This doesn't give us the license to sin. It gives us the confidence in His grace and fatherly heart. God wanst so much more for us than just to sustain us or even give us instruction. He sees us as royalty. We are children to the greatest champion of all. We are heirs to all His goodness. His words give us life and make us a chosen generation.

Prayer

Father, it can be hard sometimes to follow Your word and instruction for me, but I know that with the help of the Holy Spirit, He will guide me into all truth. Give me the understanding of the words that proceed out of Your mouth so that I can remain in right standing with You. Let the words of my mouth and meditation of my heart be acceptable in Your sight.

Exercise: Day 8

Movements	Sets	Repetitions	Rest
Burpees	3	5-10	15sec
Reverse Crunch	3	10-20	15sec
Crunch	3	10-15	1 minute than repeat

Each workout should be done in order with the given amount of rest in between. After the first set of each movement, rest for 1 minute and repeat the cycle of exercise movements. If you want to challenge yourself do more repetitions.

Visit https://www.iammetamorfit.com/21-day-journey for workouts

Journal Your Day

Day 9

Yes, I Can!

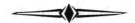

I Am *healed now by the*
stripes of Jesus Christ

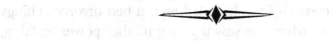

Yes, I Can!

I can do all things through Christ which strengtheneth me.

Philippians 4:13 (KJV)

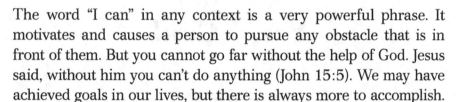

The word "I can" in any context is a very powerful phrase. It motivates and causes a person to pursue any obstacle that is in front of them. But you cannot go far without the help of God. Jesus said, without him you can't do anything (John 15:5). We may have achieved goals in our lives, but there is always more to accomplish. This is why we need God to lead us and direct us. You need His strength and His guidance.

From childhood, Laticia was told that the meaning of her name is joyful, happy and gladness. As an adult, her life seemed to be without those qualities. It started by running with the wrong crowd and making careless choices. It ended with a bad divorce. Things started to improve when she saw a young mother power walking, pushing a stroller and wearing a t-shirt that said, "I can – I WILL!" That attitude had become Laticia's personal motto to push hard, not accept bad outcomes and create the future she wanted. Yet deep down she knew she was still wounded. A friend gently, yet clearly, helped her consider that Jesus' grace was the only thing that could give her pure happiness. Today Laticia wears a t-shirt with her personal message, "I am healed – Yes, I can!"

"I can do all things through Christ," says that no matter what obstacle I face or decision I make I will not do it on my own because God is with me. God wants us to step out on faith to see our goals manifest. God leads us to places that may seem uncomfortable to us, but those are the places where God is glorified and we see His strength. Let us build our faith in this way, and know that we can do all things through Christ because He strengthens us.

Prayer

Father, I thank You that I don't have to achieve alone those things which seem hard to me. I know that through Christ Jesus, I can do it. Sometimes, I feel like giving up on my dreams and the plans you have for me, but I know that I can do all things according to Your Word. Father, You give the confidence through Your Word to go forward and never backward. Father. I pray that everything that I do, I do for Your glory and Your honor.

Exercise: Day 9

Movement	Sets	Repetitions	Rest
Running in Place	4	15-20	15sec
Burpees	4	5-15	15sec
Mountain Climbers	4	10-20	15sec
Push-ups	4	10-20	1 minute than repeat

Each workout should be done in order with the given amount of rest in between. After the first set of each movement, rest for 1 minute and repeat the cycle of exercise movements. If you want to challenge yourself do more repetitions.

Visit https://www.iammetamorfit.com/21-day-journey for workouts

_____

_____

_____

_____

_____

_____

_____

_____

_____

_____

_____

_____

_____

_____

_____

_____

_____

_____

_____

_____

_____

_____

_____

_____

_____

_____

_____

_____

_____

_____

_____

_____

Day 10

Freedom Lives in Me

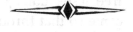

I Am loved by God
I Am saved by grace
I Am seated in heavenly
places in Chirst Jesus

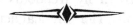

Freedom Lives in Me

**Now the Lord is the Spirit, and where the
Spirit of the Lord is, there is freedom.**

2 Corinthians 3:17 (ESV)

There is freedom in knowing who you are, and it is the Spirit of the Lord that makes you free. Jesus didn't just come so that we can make it into heaven; He came so that through Him we may know the true and living God. He came so that the relationship between God and man can be restored. Jesus became the ultimate sacrifice so that we can live free in Him.

Scottsdale Christian Academy soccer player Dasha Kem was born in Russia. Both of her biological parents died when she was just a young child, and she was placed in an orphanage deep in Siberia. In 2003, a Christian couple in Arizona adopted her. Ever since the adoption, Dasha enjoyed many freedoms and became an active member in her community. Her physical activity as a soccer player reflects how naturally the human spirit thrives with freedom. Yet, for total freedom it required her to overcome challenges and to officially pursue U.S. citizenship. In 2017, she took the oath. For her and her family it was a day to celebrate.

It is our duty as believers to glorify God in the way we live so that others may see love, truth, and the goodness of God. When we live according to God's Word, we live a life free of doubt. There might be situations in our lives that may seem harder than others, but know that there is nothing too hard for God. So, where is the Spirit of the Lord? He is in us. Therefore, we are free. We are free from doubt, free from fear, free from every ailment that holds us back from getting closer to the truth of who God is. Like Dasha, we can celebrate when we're adopted into freedom and proclaim our total citizenship in Christ. Then we can say, "freedom lives in me".

Prayer

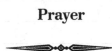

Father, I thank You that I no longer live in doubt because you have freed me through Your Son, Jesus. I thank You, Father, that You sent the comforter Holy Spirit to dwell in me so that I can walk in freedom. Help me to understand what Jesus accomplished on the cross so that I will never fall into doubt again but know that I now have the mind of Christ through His Spirit.

Exercise: Day 10

Movement	Sets	Repetitions	Rest
Front Squats	4	30 sec	10 sec
Running in place	4	30 sec	10 sec
Flutter kicks	4	30 sec	10 sec
Planks	4	30-60sec	1 minute and repeat

Each workout should be done in order with the given amount of rest in between. After the first set of each movement, rest for 1 minute and repeat the cycle of exercise movements. If you want to challenge yourself do more repetitions.

Visit https://www.iammetamorfit.com/21-day-journey for workouts

Journal Your Day

Day 11

The Battle of the Mind

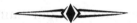

I Am more than a conqueror in Christ Jesus
Romans 8:37

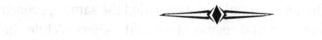

The Battle of the Mind

**For the desires of the flesh are against the Spirit,
and the desires of the Spirit are against the flesh,
for these are opposed to each other, to keep
you from doing the things you want to do.**

Galatians 5:17

Life can often seem to be a continuous tug of war between our will and God's will. We often feed our human nature and selfish desires with things that do not please God. They give us a sense of temporary pleasure and satisfaction. That is not God's will.

Samantha, had built a reputation of being a problem solver. She was decisive at work. She knew the processes of her industry and had an impressive ability to get the job done with laser focus and aggressive speed. In her personal life, she applied the same approach to her workouts, finances and relationships with others. While she usually got her way and achieved outcomes that on the surface most thought were desirable, deep down she knew that she was her own worst enemy. Those who knew her well knew of the damage she had done --- she struggled with her weight, had an unbearable load of debt and intentionally manipulated many of her friendships. Her mother had raised her well-versed in the admonition, "Do unto others as you'd have them do unto you." Samantha, long ago had devised her own interpretation of that scripture. Lately, it was getting much harder to maintain the focused and aggressive reputation.

Doing the will of God is usually uncomfortable to our self-will. In Mark's account of Jesus praying in the garden and anticipating his crucifixion, Jesus asks His Father to **"take away this cup from me: nevertheless not what I will, but what thou wilt"** Mark 14:36 (KJV). Jesus then goes on to say in verse thirty-eight that **"...the spirit truly is ready, but the flesh is weak."** When your mind argues for logic and resists the leading of God's spirit, you are out of agreement with God. That will get you nowhere. But, when our relationship with God becomes a priority in our lives, choosing God's will be our default action even when we feel uncomfortable. We should spend more time with God rather than the problem that is in front of us.

Prayer

—————◦————

Father, I thank You that on the cross Jesus overcame the flesh, and I no longer have to battle against the flesh. It is hard to discern between Your will and my will. Holy Spirit, shine a light on the truth of God's Word so that I may follow His plan for my life. Father, I have been living according to the carnal mind for too long, and it is time to completely submit my ways unto You. I know that I may have to let some people go and surround myself with people that are in Your will. Father, lead me to those who are in Your will so that I can learn from them. This may be uncomfortable for me but, Holy Spirit, You are my comforter. I trust Your leading according to God's Word.

Exercise: Day 11

Movement	Sets	Repetitions	Rest
Burpees	3	10-15	15sec
V-ups	3	10-20	15sec

| Side planks L-side | 3 | 30-45sec | 1 minute and repeat |
| Side planks R-side | | | |

Each workout should be done in order with the given amount of rest in between. After the first set of each movement, rest for 1 minute and repeat the cycle of exercise movements. If you want to challenge yourself do more repetitions.

Visit https://www.iammetamorfit.com/21-day-journey for workouts

Journal Your Day

Day 12

I'm on the Winning Side

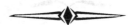

*I Am redeemed by the blood of Jesus Christ
I Am forgiven of my sins
according to his grace*

Ephesians 1:7

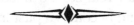

I'm on the Winning Side

We use God's mighty weapons, not worldly weapons, to knock down the strongholds of human reasoning and to destroy false arguments .We destroy every proud obstacle that keeps people from knowing God. We capture their rebellious thoughts and teach them to obey Christ.

2 Corinthians 10:4-5

Have you heard the expression, "Don't ever bring a knife to a gun fight?" Well, that can be true when you are fighting a spiritual battle. We can't take on a spiritual battle with the carnal mind. When we understand that we abide in Christ and Christ in us, we know the battle is already won.

The movie, *The Masked Saint,* tells the story of Chris Samuels (in real life, Chris Whaley) played by Brett Granstaff. Chris, a professional wrestler and family man realizes he needs something more. He retires from wrestling and becomes a pastor in a small town. Turns out, the wrestling battles are minor in comparison to the troubles he has at church. There are persistent challenges with the congregation leading to a decline in attendance and revenue. At the same time, the church is in big need of repair. Surprisingly, his wrestling skills give him the ability to defend a local resident who is being assaulted. Thus, his past starts to play a role in his present, now as a masked wrestler winning fights and raising funds for the church. He starts to find that preaching and wrestling might be a perfect match.

A wrestling match as we know it today typically only takes a few minutes to end, and a winner is declared at the end after three seconds. It took Jesus three years to accomplish a battle that we are still fighting, and it took these three winning words to declare that the battle is over on the cross "It is finished." However, when we understand that we are victorious through the blood of Jesus Christ then the wrestling match that we are fighting can be over in a matter of minutes.

Chris, the Masked Saint, learns this lesson and discovers how to be fit for God's use. As you become Metamorfit you'll find that the winning side isn't found by wrestling with God but rather in the strength you gain as you surrender to Him.

Prayer

Father, I thank You for sending Your Son, Jesus, to fight a battle that I was never prepared for. Thank You, Father, for encouraging me through your word and allowing me to see and understand that my weapon of choice is not carnal but mighty through You. Your Spirit is mighty for us. Father, let the words of Jesus Christ, "It is finished" ring louder in my ears than any other voice of discouragement. Father, I believe that what Jesus Christ did on the cross was enough to win that battle that I am currently wrestling with. I understand now that the battle was never mine to begin with. It was Your battle and You have won. Now, I am victorious.

Exercise: Day 12

Movements	Sets	Repetitions	Rest
Russian Twist	4	10-20	15sec
Sitting Crunches	4	10-20	15sec

Mountain Climbers	4	10-20	15sec
Planks	4	20-45	15sec

Each workout should be done in order with the given amount of rest in between. After the first set of each movement, rest for 1 minute and repeat the cycle of exercise movements. If you want to challenge yourself do more repetitions.

Visit https://www.iammetamorfit.com/21-day-journey for workouts

Journal Your Day

Day 13

What have you Given Birth To?

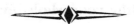

I Am the temple of God
I belong to God
1 Corinthians 6:19

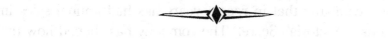

What have you Given Birth To?

**Humans can reproduce only human life, but
the Holy Spirit gives birth to spiritual life.**

John 3:6 (NLT)

Jesus said in Matthew 6:22 (NLT),

**"Your eye is like a lamp that provides light for your body.
When your eye is healthy, your whole body is filled with light."**

Like David, the author of the Psalm, we should work daily not to set
any wicked thing before our eyes. It's easy to convince ourselves that
the things of this world will not harm us. However, when we embrace
the perspective that we are the temple of the Holy Spirit then we
must invite into our spirit only those things that are pleasing to God.

You may not know Roy Raymond, but on June 12, 1977, he gave
birth to a company that in recent years has had annual sales in
the billions – Victoria's Secret. The company has shaped how the
world sees women and how women view themselves. To be selected
as a Victoria's Secret Angel and model the brand to the world is
considered a rare honor in the modeling industry. Kylie Bisutti
achieved that distinction and fed a growing and successful career.

Along the way God helped her to change directions. She says, "The
Lord graciously opened my eyes and saved me from the love of
worldliness that was taking me over. He brought me to a place in

my life of realization and truth! He reshaped my desires for my life and showed me that my body is a temple and was created to be honoring to Him in all things, especially in my marriage and in being an example to younger girls!"

When we invite the things of this world into our lives, we conceive the things of the flesh. That gives birth to a way of life that models worldliness and overtime leads us away from the beautiful vision of what God has designed for each of us. When Jesus went to the cross, He overcame the world by taking the sins upon His flesh.

When we remain in God's Word and continue to communicate with God through prayer, we will continue to feed our spiritual man and give birth to the things of the Spirit. Let us hold fast to the things that were birthed through the Spirit by embracing God's Word and not the things that were birthed through the flesh by man.

Prayer

Father, forgive me for pursuing things that You never invited into this temple. Father, my flesh sometimes lusts after the things of the flesh, and not the things of the Spirit. I ask that you cut from the root those wicked things that I allowed into my soul. Show me those things I must let go so that I will birth the things of the Spirit. Help me to be aware of the things that are born of the flesh and out of the Spirit so that I can be fed properly. Cleanse me through Your Word. Your Word is true.

Exercise: Day 13

Movements	Sets	Repetitions	Rest
Running in Place	4	10-20	No Rest
Burpees	4	10-15	No Rest
Mountain Climbers	4	10-15	1 minute repeat

Each workout should be done in order with the given amount of rest in between. After the first set of each movement, rest for 1 minute and repeat the cycle of exercise movements. If you want to challenge yourself do more repetitions.

Visit https://www.iammetamorfit.com/21-day-journey for workouts

Journal Your Day

_____

_____

_____

_____

_____

_____

_____

_____

_____

_____

_____

_____

_____

_____

_____

_____

_____

_____

_____

_____

_____

_____

_____

_____

_____

_____

_____

_____

_____

_____

_____

_____

_____

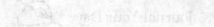

Day 14

"But God, everyone is doing it."

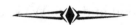

I Am *born again through the word*
of God through Jesus Christ

1 Peter1:23

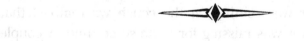

"But God, everyone is doing it."

With the Lord's authority I say this: Live no longer as the Gentiles do, for they are hopelessly confused.

Ephesians 4:17(ESV)

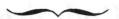

Before the written Word of God, men and women tried to live by the words that proceeded out of the mouth of God. God, in the beginning, said to Adam in Genesis 2:17 that they would die if they ate of the tree of good and evil. We know that Adam and Eve didn't exactly die a physical death, but it was a spiritual death that they experienced through the lust of the eyes and disobedience. This caused separation from God which could be considered the spiritual death.

My young daughter has a sweet tooth just like her mother and will try her best to get to the Easter candy hidden in the closet or the cupcakes that are on top of the counter. One day while my wife and eldest daughter were sitting on the couch we realized that my youngest daughter was missing for quite some time. A couple of minutes after realizing that she was gone, I called for her. She quickly ran back to the living room licking her fingers with the residue of red velvet cupcake all over her mouth.

I wasn't very happy with what she had done. However, the discipline of the moment wasn't about me it was about helping her to grow. She wasn't allowed to have any more cupcake for the rest of the day.

Children, like my daughter, at the formative age of three are very smart and want to learn from mommy and daddy.

When we walk after the things of the flesh, we will always be separated from God's will and purpose. But if we mortify or discipline the body when we are faced with the temptation of the flesh, then we will live an abundant life given by Jesus.

Prayer

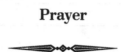

Father, help me not to walk in the ways of the world, in the vanity of the mind. Show me daily through Your Word the way I must walk. Help me to be aware of my actions that do not glorify You and teach me to have self-control so that Your light will shine.

Exercise: Day 14

Movement	Sets	Repetitions	Rest
Jumping Squats	4	10-15	15 sec
Power-ups	4	10-15	15sec
Planks	4	60-90sec	45 sec repeat

Each workout should be done in order with the given amount of rest in between. After the first set of each movement, rest for 1 minute and repeat the cycle of exercise movements. If you want to challenge yourself do more repetitions.

Visit https://www.iammetamorfit.com/21-day-journey for workouts

Journal Your Day

Day 15

Am I Condemned?

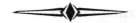

*I **Am** a Child of God, according to his Spirit*

Romans 8:16

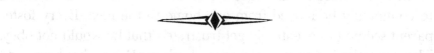

Am I Condemned?

**There is therefore now no condemnation to
them which are in Christ Jesus, who walk not
after the flesh, but after the Spirit.**

Romans 8:1 (KJV)

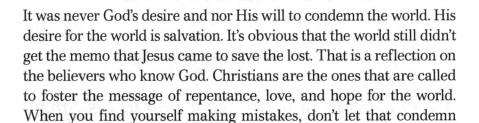

It was never God's desire and nor His will to condemn the world. His desire for the world is salvation. It's obvious that the world still didn't get the memo that Jesus came to save the lost. That is a reflection on the believers who know God. Christians are the ones that are called to foster the message of repentance, love, and hope for the world. When you find yourself making mistakes, don't let that condemn you, instead get back up and keep walking.

Jason is a fourteen-year-old foster child who felt he was destined to continually be moved from one home to the next. Every foster parent seemed to eventually get frustrated that he would not obey. That led to bad feelings, tempers and yelling. When that happened Jason usually found himself alone in his room, hopeless and crying until he fell asleep.

The Martinez family was different. They didn't yell at him for doing wrong. Instead they helped him to do better, so that he could learn from his mistakes and mature as a young man. One night after dinner Jason retreated quickly to his room to resume playing a new video game. Two hours later his foster mother came to him and asked him to come down stairs. Back in the dining room he saw that the dishes were still on the table, waiting for him to clean them as he had agreed to do.

Jason began to cry, but this time for a different reason. He realized he had a new destiny. He was being given the opportunity to be part of the family. His foster mother comforted him and told him that she prayed for him often and was proud to see him taking greater ownership of his potential and being responsible. Jason quickly wiped his tears, got to work and said, "Thanks, I needed that". With time Jason found he cried less and had more reasons to be thankful for the changes God was doing in his life.

Condemnation comes from the world. When your thinking is clouded by selfishness, hopelessness and lies and you fail to embrace the things of God, then you are condemned already. The world has a new chance each day to know God through faithful missionaries around the world – Christians who have had a life change and share the joy and power of that transformation with others. Romans 1:19 says, "It was made plain to them because God has shown it to them." We know, through God's word, what is right and profitable. So, choose today to walk after the Spirit's leading. Share God's ways with others and help them to be metamorfit.

Prayer

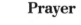

Father, I thank You that Your love reaches far past me. You have given me an opportunity to walk after Your Spirit. I know I make mistakes and fall short. I also know that You will never condemn me because I believe in Your Son, Jesus Christ. I know that when I do feel condemnation that it is coming from another source. Help me, through your Word, to see what I lack so that I can continue to walk as light for the world to see.

Exercise: Day 15

Movement	Sets	Repetitions	Rest
Mountain Climbers	7	7	No rest
Push-ups	7	7	No rest

Each workout should be done in order with the given amount of rest in between. After the first set of each movement, rest for 1 minute and repeat the cycle of exercise movements. If you want to challenge yourself do more repetitions.

Visit https://www.iammetamorfit.com/21-day-journey for workouts

Journal Your Day

Day 16

Transformed from Distraction to Mission

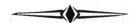

*I Am not condemned, because
I Am in Christ Jesus*

Romans 8:1

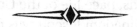

Transformed from
Distraction to Mission

**For the world offers only a craving for physical
pleasure, a craving for everything we see, and pride
in our achievements and possessions. These are
not from the Father, but are from this world.**

1 John 2:16(NLT)

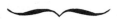

Jesus says that we are in this world but not of it. That means, even though a world full of comforts, must-have items, entertainment and other flashy things beg for our attention and investment, we can live surrounded by the flashy things of this world as children of God. We live according to the kingdom.

Joseph Sagawa a transfer student from Uganda was recruited to play professional soccer in the UK. Joseph grew up in a very poor village and wasn't used to the fast pace life of the United Kingdom. During his tour of the United Kingdom Joseph was placed in a 5 star hotel with the finest of amenities. The plush hotel bed was bigger than the room of his home in Uganda where he and his three brothers all slept on mats. Joseph spread the sheets on the floor, creating a space to which he was accustomed, and slept comfortably there the whole night. The next morning when the recruiter arrived he noticed that Joseph had slept on the floor. The recruiter asked him why he chose to sleep there rather than the premium hotel bed. Joseph said that in his culture being comfortable is not determined by how much you have, but who you are. Material things will never change who I am.

Followers of Christ, shouldn't allow material things to be their goal – to be the things that satisfy them more than God. Those who don't embrace this Christian perspective will always push for more worldly comforts and temporary satisfactions. That's not what motivated Jesus. Christ was satisfied with doing the will of His Father. He had a mission to accomplish here on earth, and He didn't allow the things of this world, even the good things of this world, to distract Him. A Christian worldview compels you to pursue God and fulfill your mission on earth, realizing that *the pursuit* of comforts is what distracts and puts you off course. We do the will of God by daily continuing in His instruction and leading. Jesus' words are enduring and become powerful in our lives when we openly receive them. When you understand and embrace the mission that God gives you, it should compel and drive your passion more than the distractions. So, what does God call you to do?

Prayer

———⟫◆⟪———

Father, forgive me when I allow the things of this world to be first in my life and not You. My intentions are to serve You, Father. However, there are so many distractions. Father, I ask that You show me those things that I need to let go of in order to have more time with You. I know You have called me to do a mission, but I need Your guidance on applying the vision You have given to me. Help me live according to the Kingdom of heaven and not by the kingdoms of this world. Transform my desires that I can be metamorfit.

Exercise: Day 16

Movement	Sets	Repetitions	Rest
Jumping Jacks	5	20-30	10sec
Knee Kicks Right and Left	5	20-30 each side	10 sec
Burpee Jumps	5	10	45 sec

Journal Your Day

_____
_____
_____
_____
_____
_____
_____
_____
_____
_____
_____
_____
_____
_____
_____
_____
_____
_____
_____
_____
_____
_____
_____
_____
_____

Day 17

I Am Made New

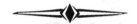

I Am made righteous in God
through Christ Jesus
2 Corinthians 5:21

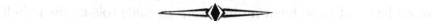

I Am Made New

But that is not the way you learned Christ!— assuming that you have heard about him and were taught in him, as the truth is in Jesus, to put off your old self, which belongs to your former manner of life and is corrupt through deceitful desires, and to be renewed in the spirit of your minds, and to put on the new self, created after the likeness of God in true righteousness and holiness.

Ephesians 4:20-24(ESV)

There are many great leaders who have come and gone. Many of them we still talk about today. We build statues of them and name holidays after them. Yet despite their good works and positive example, none of them have done what Jesus Christ has done for us.

Joe was a troubled kid. As he got older it got worse. His father left when he was ten, so he never had a strong male role model to help him become a man of character. He would hang out with other troubled youth and follow men who had money, cars, women and all the flashy things. He fell into drugs and alcohol and was locked up a few times.

Years passed and one afternoon as he was walking down the street. A tall man in a brown coat walked up to him and reached in his pocket. Joe was terrified that he would pull out a gun but was relieved to see that instead the man only held a Bible. The man then said just three words to Joe, "Jesus loves you". He gave Joe the

Bible and walked away. It had been over twenty years since Joe had heard these words, but for some reason this time it sunk deep and had real meaning.

He began reading the Bible and later gave his life to God. Shortly, thereafter, Joe once again was walking the same street to home and again a tall man with a brown coat reached in his pocket --- this time Joe was confronted with a gun pointing toward him. Joe didn't hesitate to say three words, "Jesus loves you". The tall man recognized Joe's voice and realized that Joe, the man he was confronting, was the 10-year old boy he had hung out with years ago. He offered him a beer, and Joe quickly replied, "I'm a new man." It was at that moment Joe new that he was a changed man with a spiritual fitness that God could use.

We've all been in a dark place. You may be struggling today. Jesus died so that you can put away the old person you were and through repentance and receiving Jesus Christ put on a new, life-giving nature. It is a daily process, but that is why we are sealed with the Holy Spirit. Don't try to handle your problems by yourself; you have your Heavenly Father, God, who takes care of all your worries. When you trust in your own efforts you doubt God and grieve the Holy Spirit. Continue to trust, be still and obey, then your mind will be renewed and you can walk saying, "I am made new."

Prayer

Father, I thank You that you have sent Your son to die so that I may live. Father, I sometimes struggle with the things of the past, but I know in my heart that I'm no longer that person. You have given me a better way which is Jesus Christ. Father, You make all things new, and I am new in Christ. The old has passed away, and the new has come.

Exercise: Day 17

Movement	Sets	Repetitions	Rest
Burpee Jumps	5	10-15	15sec
Side Steps	5	10	15sec
Front Squats	5	10-15	15sec
Push up Jacks	5	10-15	1 minute than repeat

Each workout should be done in order with the given amount of rest in between. After the first set of each movement, rest for 1 minute and repeat the cycle of exercise movements. If you want to challenge yourself do more repetitions.

Visit https://www.iammetamorfit.com/21-day-journey for workouts

Journal Your Day

Day 18

Are you Satisfied?

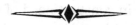

I Am transformed by the renewing of my mind according to God's word

Romans 12:2

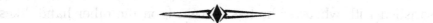

Are you Satisfied?

Let them praise the Lord for his great love and for the wonderful things he has done for them. For he satisfies the thirsty and fills the hungry with good things.

Psalm 107:8-9 (NLT)

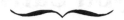

Our soul and body are in constant need of satisfaction. Sometimes we satisfy that need with things that are not pleasing to God. Maybe we might want a good laugh but feeding our mind with cruel comedy and lies may not be the best medicine. Maybe we might want a midnight snack but feeding our body with fried foods late at night might not be good for our health.

Bret and Bernard are twin teenaged boys who have different outlooks on life. Bret is the calm and humble one who is generally satisfied with whatever he has. Bernard, on the other hand, likes the finer things and tends to complain and wants or expects more.

On their sixteenth birthday they both received cars. Their parents worked really hard to make it happen and hoped that they would both love it. As Bret and Barnard went outside they were both met with a late-model Honda Accord one silver and the other blue. Bret burst into cheers of joy and hugged both his parents. Bernard on the other hand complained at the fact that they were ten years old and used. His parents explained to him that this was the only thing they could afford but gave him the choice to do whatever he wanted to do with the car.

Bernard decided to sell it and use the money toward a down payment on a new Honda Accord. What Bernard hadn't considered was that he would have to start making monthly payments. Insurance was a whole other issue. When he realized that a new car wasn't going to be within his ability, he quickly tried to get his old car back from the new owner, but that person had already sold it to a used car dealership.

A week later while riding home from school with his brother Bret, there in front of the house was the same blue Honda. Puzzled, he quickly jumped out of the car, ran to his parents and asked who owned the car now. The father replied, "Son, sometimes what you want will only leave you with more responsibilities, but what you need will keep you comfortable."

God is the only one that can satisfy our soul with everything we need. We may not understand His plan, but we know that every good and perfect thing is from above. The Holy Spirit reveals to us God's goodness and wonderful works. When we continue to stay postured in the presence of God, we will always be satisfied.

Prayer

Father, I thank You that You satisfy me with Your word and Your presence. Forgive me, Father, if I have abandoned the truth in Your word to find a quick and temporary satisfaction given by the world and not from You. Help me to understand Your goodness and Your wonderful works towards me that I may be satisfied all the days of my life. And just like David in the Bible, I pray that your goodness and mercy will follow me all the days of my life.

Exercise: Day 18

Movement	Sets	Repetitions	Rest
Jumping Jacks	5	20-30	15sec
Knee Kicks	5	10-20	15sec
Side to Side Planks	5	30 sec	1 minute than repeat

Each workout should be done in order with the given amount of rest in between. After the first set of each movement, rest for 1 minute and repeat the cycle of exercise movements. If you want to challenge yourself do more repetitions.

Visit https://www.iammetamorfit.com/21-day-journey for workouts

Journal Your Day

_____
_____
_____
_____
_____
_____
_____
_____
_____
_____
_____
_____
_____
_____
_____
_____
_____
_____
_____
_____
_____
_____
_____
_____
_____
_____
_____
_____
_____
_____

Day 19

How do you know you Love God?

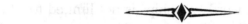

I Am nothing without Jesus Christ the Son of God
John 15:5

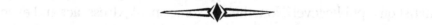

How do you know you Love God?

**"Teacher, which is the most important
commandment in the law of Moses?"
Jesus replied, "'You must love the Lord your God
with all your heart, all your soul, and all your
mind.' This is the first and greatest commandment.**

Matthew 22:36-38 (NLT)

Did you know that the word "worship" is not limited to Christian believers or someone of a religious sect? Worship is showing honor or reverence to any person, god or object. Many different people can express it in a variety of ways.

Go to a concert of a major pop star and you'll see a stadium packed with people who listen to that artist's music daily. Many try to sing like their music idol. While a few people are personal contacts with these stars, the vast majority of people will only connect with the artist on a public level. Nonetheless, some speak, dress, act and even think like their icon. Some of these people, in an attempt to better connect with that person, will even do outrageous things to their body in the name of that artist. It all seems harmless, but beyond the surface appearances it has an effect on their spirit, soul, and body.

Whether we want to admit it or not, people become gods in our lives when we give them greater importance and invest more in them than God. In fact, a good thing like self-improvement can, however unintentional, cause us to "worship" our self and distract us from God and His greater vision for us.

Jessy had been feeling very insecure about her weight and body image which led her to feel that nobody loved her. One day while sipping a lite latte with her friend in the café her friend asked a very simple but profound question, "Do you think God loves you?" Jessy said with confidence, "Yes, of course, He does". Then her friend asked, "What parts of you does He love?" Then Jessy, trying to understand what point her friend was making, ventured a guess, "All of me?" Her friend asked her, "If God loves you so much, and everything about you, shouldn't you love what God loves?" Jessy realized that she was putting greater trust in her own feelings rather than abiding in the greater confidence she has in God. It was the metamorphosis of thinking and believing that she needed to take care of her body with healthy eating and exercise. More importantly, she discovered that worshiping God was as simple as speaking healthy words, God's words, over her life every day.

In order to worship God in spirit with a pure heart, we must first honestly examine what things we put ahead of God. God has to come first in everything we do. When we love God with all of our heart, soul, and mind, we live a lifestyle of worship.

Prayer

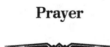

Father, You have shown me through Your Word that I must put you first and love you with my heart, soul, and mind. Father, even though I can't see You in the flesh, I know that You are there with me. So, I worship you. Father, even though I can't feel You all the time I know that You are there. So, I worship You. Father, it can be hard to focus on Your presence because of the distractions of the world. Help me learn the simplicity of worship through your word and live a lifestyle of worship so that others may follow.

Exercise: Day 19

Movements	Sets	Repetitions	Rest
Mountain Climbers	5	10-20	15sec
Crunches	5	20-30	15sec
Side Planks w/hip drop ® (L)	5	15-20	15sec
Plank	5	45-60sec	1 minute than repeat

Each workout should be done in order with the given amount of rest in between. After the first set of each movement, rest for 1 minute and repeat the cycle of exercise movements. If you want to challenge yourself do more repetitions.

Visit https://www.iammetamorfit.com/21-day-journey for workouts

Journal Your Day

_____
_____
_____
_____
_____
_____
_____
_____
_____
_____
_____
_____
_____
_____
_____
_____
_____
_____
_____
_____
_____
_____
_____
_____
_____
_____
_____
_____
_____

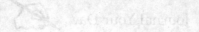

Day 20

Finding Rest in God

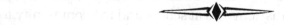

I Am God's child
I Am an over comer
I Have greatness living inside of me
1 John 4:4

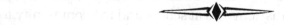

Finding Rest in God

Take my yoke upon you, and learn from me, for I am gentle and lowly in heart, and you will find rest for your souls.

Matthew 11:29 (ESV)

God blesses us with many material things. Sometimes we forget that they are only temporary. Sometimes though we're just like the rich young ruler in the Bible who found it difficult to fully follow Jesus because of these many possessions. David's prayer in the scripture is for God not to take His Spirit away from him. That should be our prayer as well.

Rick is an eighteen year old senior at a high school in Australia who is very involved at school and in the community. He is a track and field athlete, captain of the debate team, part of the backstage crew, youth leader at his church, and he also volunteers at the nursing home on weekends. Rick has been blessed with many opportunities. But, he has been using his activities at school and the community to hide an aspect of his life where he is uneasy. Rick has been bullied at school for years. He never told his father about it because he felt ashamed that he couldn't overcome the problem on his own.

When he finally did open up to his father about it and tell him, his father embraced him with a big hug and let him know that he would be there for him.

We may not be able to get everything we want or need in life. We need to learn instead to turn to God the Father and cast our concerns upon Him. God's Spirit is more precious than anything in this world. It is His Spirit that leads us to a place of rest for our souls. Jesus says that when we learn of Him we can find rest for our souls. Jesus wants to give us rest, but we must allow Him to guide and direct us. This is why we need the Holy Spirit; He teaches us the way of meekness and lowliness.

Prayer

Father, I am not at a place where all I want is Your presence in my life, but I know that your Spirit is what guides me through your Word and reveals the true nature and character of Jesus. Give me a clean heart, Father, and renew a right Spirit within me. Search my heart and see if there be any wickedness in me. Show me if I have been bitter, prideful or unforgiving. Father, search the deep things of my spirit. Help me to become meek and lowly in the heart so that I may find rest for my soul.

Exercise: Day 20

Movements	Sets	Repetitions	Rest
Burpee Jumps	5	10-15	15sec
Elevated push-ups	5	10-20	15sec
Reverse crunches	5	10-25	15sec

Each workout should be done in order with the given amount of rest in between. After the first set of each movement, rest for 1 minute and repeat the cycle of exercise movements. If you want to challenge yourself do more repetitions.

Visit https://www.iammetamorfit.com/21-day-journey for workouts

Journal Your Day

Day 21

God's Powerful Word

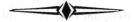

I Am a friend of Jesus

God's Powerful Word

For the word of God is alive and powerful. It is sharper than the sharpest two-edged sword, cutting between soul and spirit, between joint and marrow. It exposes our innermost thoughts and desires.

Hebrews 4:12 (NLT)

Growing up I have always admired my father. I still do. He is the only man after whom I model my life. Friends and family that know us say things like, "You are just like your father," or "You sound like daddy." It's true – I can't deny it.

A perfect stranger, on the other hand, may look at my patient nature or respectful demeanor and give all the credit to me. They would never know that I had a proper upbringing by an upright man. They might only see the results of what I was taught through the years by my father on how to be a man.

God sent His Son not only to save the world but to be a model for the world. How can the world receive a truth that can't be seen? God puts His Spirit in Christians so that they can live the life of love, truth, peace and hope for those that don't have it. The only way the world will know about a Heavenly Father is if Christians live a transformed life according to His holy Word and be the very essence of what it means to be metamorfit. A Christian's intent should be to model God in every way. God's Word is powerful. It empowers us to see the world according to His heart and desire – and then to look and sound just like Him. God's powerful Word, alive in Christians, can be the hope for those that are seeking the truth.

Prayer

Father, I thank You that You have never left me nor forsaken me. You have been with me the whole time. Lord, I want to be a vessel that demonstrates Your love to the world. I want to be a vessel that carries out the truth of Jesus Christ and bring hope to a dying world. I will live out Your Word with joy and gladness that the world may see You and not me. Father, continue to sanctify me through Your Word for Your Word is true.

Exercise: Day 21

Movements	Sets	Repetitions	Rest
Burpees	5	10-15	No rest
Mountain Climbers	5	10-20	No rest
Push-ups	5	10-15-30	No rest
V-ups	5	10-20	1minute rest repeat

Each workout should be done in order with the given amount of rest in between. After the first set of each movement, rest for 1 minute and repeat the cycle of exercise movements. If you want to challenge yourself do more repetitions.

Visit https://www.iammetamorfit.com/21-day-journey for workouts

Journal Your Day

This is just the Beginning

I wouldn't call this a "conclusion," but the beginning of a lifestyle that you can pass on to your friends and family. You have been given knowledge through this book. Apply it to your life and don't keep it to yourself. Take what you have learned from your journey through journaling, exercising, and prayer and teach others. Be diligent in God's Word; praying on a daily basis. Continue to do more research on health and fitness. Learn other ways to maintain a steady and healthy life.

Be mindful of the foods you put in your body and how many times you work out in a day. You may have a busy life and may not have enough time to work out, but try to make some sacrifices; your body deserves it. You are God's creation. He gives you and no one else the responsibility to be a good steward and take care of you.

My prayer is that God will continue to guide you through the next part of your journey. Be looking. He will place other people in your life that have a desire to live physically and spiritually healthy. I pray that God will teach you how to be patient with the process and not get frustrated. Trust that God will honor every step you take and every move you make toward your goal. Eagerly look for the transformation. Anticipate the beautiful change that only God can miraculously orchestrate. It happens when you pursue Him daily to get metamorfit. God bless you.

This is just the Beginning

Acknowledgements

I just want to thank all those that supported me in this new journey. God has placed this vision in my heart, unexpectedly, and it was a bit outside of my comfort zone. But many of you have prayed and sowed into my life. To my mother and father Donald and Sharon Stevens, thank you for supporting me through prayers and your love. To my three amazing sisters: Camille Holmes, Christine and Alexandria Stevens, thank you for your love and support and believing in this vision that God has given me. I want to give a special thanks to Daniel Josephs and Darryl Davis for being my right hand man throughout this project. To those who supported me financially-thank you, Alina, Mina, Alexandria, Donna, Rafael, Darryl, Nathan, Kevin, Francis, Jeremy, Rick, Akintunde, Quar-an, Israel, Camille, Dontrell, Daniel A., Gregory, Ari, Jason, Brad, Randy, Craig, Leighton, Krystal, Tahira, Lynn, Antonio, Narda, Freedom, Larry, Garnett, Keara and Hubert, Sonia C, Cassandra. V, Maria. G, Pauline, Neal,

I could not have done this without your financial support, and I pray God will give you back everything and more that you have sown. I also want to thank Jermaine Haughton of **Jermaine Haughton Photography** for the pictures, EJAE the Entertainer of **Baritone Design Studio** for the cover design. And last, but not least, to my lovely wife and three beautiful girls. To my wife Arsenia, you have stuck with me through all the discouragement and sad times. Thank you so much for your unconditional love and support. Babe, I love you with all my heart. And to my two beautiful girls Gabby and Saniyah, thank you allowing daddy to do God's work. I love you.

Thank you all and may God continue to bless you even more.

About the Author

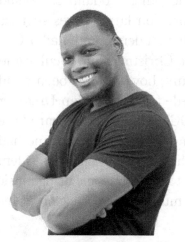

Donald L Stevens Jr is a devoted Christian who believes that Jesus Christ is the only way to everlasting life. He cherishes the words of God and is a student of the word. Donald not only studies the word, but is a doer of the word, and believes that God's word is living and active, but we must walk in it. Donald is a father of two girls Saniyah and Gabriella Stevens, and husband of one wife Arsenia Stevens. Donald is devoted to making his girls happy and leading by a good example they way Christ has intended. Donald currently lives in White Plains, NY where he was born and raised by his two parents Donald Sr and Sharon Stevens, joined by his three sisters Camille, Christine and Alex.

Donald L Stevens Jr has been preaching the gospel of Jesus Christ since 2008, and has equipped churches and other ministries to impact their community and surrounding areas. Donald has seen many miracles and healings happen through this ministry and many have come to know the Lord as their personal savior. In June of 2017 he led over thirty missionaries from different states on a evangelistic event in New York City where they saw God move in powerful way through song, dance, testimony, and preaching love and repentance to non-believers. His desire is to see many lives touched by the power of the gospel with signs following. Donald continues to impact his community and other surrounding areas with the gospel message.

Donald has received his Masters degree in Music Therapy from New York University, and currently serves over 200 children and adults with disabilities in Westchester, NY. Through music Donald has seen many children and adults overcome obstacles that used to be a hindrance for since birth, and they continue to progress every year through music therapy and other modalities. Donald was graced with opportunity to perform on large stages such as Madison Square Garden twice with his students, and Radio City Music Hall where he opened up for the Christmas Spectacular and performed a song he wrote with a young boy who has been blind from birth. Donald was recently awarded the American Dreamer Award from Southern Westchester BOCES. Donald has shared the same stage with Grammy Award Winner Israel Haughton, and had the opportunity to play behind Evangelist Daniel Kolenda, President of Christ for Nations. Donald continues to impact people using music in school, and in church as the head musician and Deacon at his church.

Donald is former 2 time All-American in track and field from Southern Connecticut State University where he received his Bachelors of Arts in Music and honored at the Convocation as being one the top students in the department of music. Donald had hopes of running in the 2016 Olympics but came to a standstill after suffering from a pulled hamstring and injured back. After a dry season of not working out, and eating unhealthy, Donald gained forty pounds and felt the effects of his weight with sharp pains in chest, and not being able to carry his own weight. He decided it was time to get serious about his health and started working out again. Donald learned how to balance his eating by going vegan for a few months and learned the benefits of eating raw foods, and eating in moderation. The gym became his second home, and when he wasn't in the gym he made it his priority to work out at home. He started coaching others who wanted to lose weight, get stronger, and have an overall great health physically as well as spiritually. He began to see results of the effort they have put in, and decided to work with people voluntarily. Since then, people have grown strong physically and spiritually. Donald continues to inspire people all over with faith and fitness.

Printed in the United States
By Bookmasters